Benefits Of Aloe Vera

Tammie Rowe

ISBN: 9798555194817

Contents

ACKNOWLEDGMENTS

Aloe vera is a medicinal plant that's been used to treat various health conditions for thousands of years. It's usually safe to use also vera directly from the plant or you can buy it in gel form.

Aloe vera creams, gels, and ointments contain the clear gel found in aloe veraleaves. These products can be applied topically to treat various skin conditions. Aloe is sold in capsule or liquid form to take internally to promote health and well-being.

Read on to learn how to use aloe vera and the potential benefits and risks.

1.HOW TO HARVEST THE PLANT

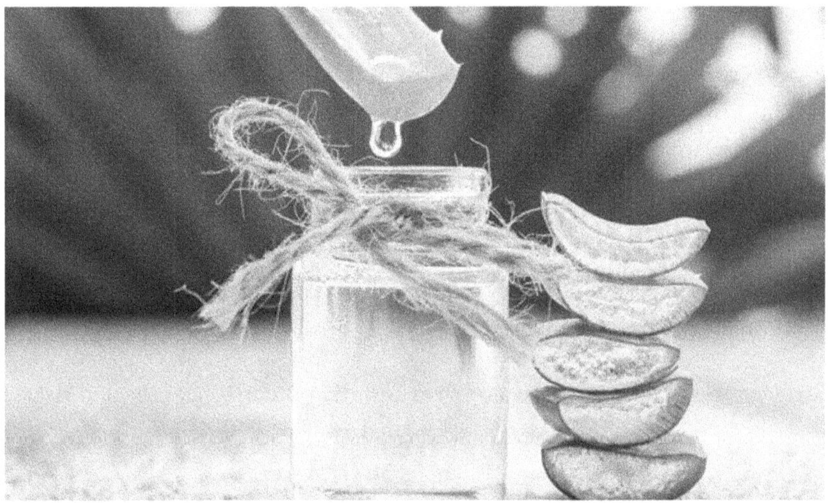

It's relatively simple to harvest an aloe plant for gel and juice. You'll need a mature plant that's at least a few years old. This ensures a higher concentration of the active ingredients.

You'll also want to wait a few weeks before cutting leaves from the same plant. You may want to have a few plants on rotation if you plan to harvest aloe often.

To harvest your aloe plant for gel and juice:

1. Remove 3-4 leaves at a time, choosing thick leaves from the outer sections of the plant.

2. Ensure the leaves are healthy and free of any mold or damage.

3. Cut them close to the stem. Most of the beneficial nutrients are found at the base of the leaves.

4. Avoid the roots.

5. Wash and dry the leaves.

6. Trim the prickly edges with a knife.

7. Using a knife or your fingers, separate the interior gel from the outside of the leaf. The interior gel is the part of the aloe that you'll use.

8. Allow the yellow sap to drain from the leaf. This is the aloe vera latex. If you plan to use the latex, you can catch this in a container. If you're not planning to use the latex, you can dispose of it.

9. Cut the aloe gel into slices or cubes.

If you want smooth aloe gel, after separating the aloe from the exterior part of the leaf, you can put the aloe into a blender and then strain the substance to remove the pulp.

How to use fresh aloe gel

You can apply fresh aloe gel directly to your skin or follow a recipe to make a homemade beauty product. It can also be added to food, smoothies, and drinks.

To make aloe juice, use 1 cup of liquid for every 2 tablespoons of aloe gel. Include any other ingredients, like fruit, and use a blender or food processor to mix up your drink.

If you're planning to consume the fresh slices of aloe gel, it will keep in the refrigerator for a few days, but its best to consume it as quickly as possible. You can always store aloe vera gel in the freezer if you're not ready to use it right away.

9 Healthy Benefits of Drinking Aloe Vera Juice

What is aloe vera juice?

The aloe vera plant is a succulent plant species from the genus *Aloe*. It grows abundantly in tropical climates and has been used for centuries as a medicinal plant.

Aloe vera juice is a gooey, thick liquid made from the flesh of the aloe vera plant leaf. It's commonly known to treat sunburns. But drinking this healthy elixir in juice form provides you with a number of other health benefits.

Aloe vera juice is made by crushing or grinding the entire leaf of the aloe vera plant, followed by various steps to purify and filter the liquid. With a mild, tolerable flavor, the juice mixes easily into smoothies and shakes. This makes aloe vera juice a practical whole food supplement.

What are the health benefits of drinking aloe vera juice?

Here are eight reasons to drink pure, uncolored, low anthraquinone aloe vera juice.

1. Hydration

The aloe plant is very water-dense, so it's an ideal way to prevent or treat dehydration. Staying hydrated helps your body detox by providing a way for you to purge and flush out impurities. The juice also packs a hefty punch of nutrients that optimize your body's organ output.

This is crucial, because your kidneys and liver are largely responsible for the task of detoxifying your blood and producing urine. For this reason, you need to keep them healthy.

Recovery from heavy exercise also requires rehydration through the intake of extra fluids. Your body requires more fluids in order to flush and rid itself of the lactic acid buildup from exercising. Try aloe vera juice instead of coconut water after your next hard workout.

2. Liver function

When it comes to detoxing, healthy liver function is key.

Aloe vera juice is an excellent way to keep your liver healthy. That's because the liver functions best when the body is adequately nourished and hydrated. Aloe vera juice is ideal for the liver because it's hydrating and rich in phytonutrients.

3. For constipation

Drinking aloe vera juice helps increase the water content in your intestines. Research has shown a relationship between increasing the intestinal water content and the stimulation of peristalsis, which helps you pass stool normally.

If you're constipated or have problems with frequent constipation, try incorporating aloe vera juice into your daily routine. Aloe also helps normalize the healthy bacteria in your gut, keeping your healthy intestinal flora balanced.

4. For clear skin

Hydrating aloe vera juice may help reduce the frequency and appearance of acne.It may also help reduce skin conditions like psoriasis and dermatitis.

Aloe vera is a rich source of antioxidants and vitamins that may help protect your skin.

The important compounds in aloe vera have also been shown to neutralize the effects of ultraviolet (UV) radiation, repair your skin from existing UV damage, and help prevent fine lines and wrinkles.

5. Nutritious boost

Aloe vera juice is jam-packed with nutrients. Drinking it is an excellent way to make sure you don't become deficient. It contains important vitamins and minerals like vitamins B, C, E, and folic acid.

It also contains small amounts of:

- calcium

- copper

- chromium

- sodium

- selenium

- magnesium

- potassium

- manganese

- zinc

Aloe vera is one of the only plant sources of vitamin B-12, too. This is excellent news for vegetarians and vegans.

Keeping your food and drink intake nutrient-rich is key in combating most preventable diseases.

6. Heartburn relief

Drinking aloe vera juice may give you relief when heartburn attacks. The compounds present in aloe vera juice help control secretion of acid in your stomach. The effects have even been shown to combat gastric ulcers and keep them from getting larger.

7. Digestive benefits

Aloe vera contains several enzymes known to help in the breakdown of sugars and fats and to keep your digestion running smoothly.

If your digestive system isn't operating optimally, you won't absorb all of the nutrients from the food you're eating. You have to keep your internal engine healthy in order to reap the benefits from your diet.

Aloe vera may help decrease irritation in the stomach and intestines. The juice may also help people with irritable bowel syndrome (IBS) and other inflammatory disorders of the intestines.

One 2013 study of 33 IBS patients found that aloe vera juice helped reduce the pain and discomfort of IBS. The studyTrusted Source was not placebo-controlled, so more research is needed.

Aloe vera was also beneficial to people suffering from ulcerative colitis in an earlier double-blind, placebo-controlled study.

8. Beauty hacks

Keeping aloe vera juice on hand can also be good for a number of beauty and health needs.

Try using it for the following:

- makeup primer (apply before foundation)

- makeup remover

- sunburn soother

- lightweight moisturizer

- treatment for irritated scalp (mix in a few drops of peppermint oil)

What are the side effects of drinking aloe vera juice?

Decolorized (purified, low anthraquinone) whole leaf aloe vera is considered safe. A 2013 study in mice fed various concentrations of purified aloe vera for three months showed no adverse effects at all from the juice.

Colored vs. decolorized aloe juice

On the other hand, nondecolorized, unpurified aloe vera juice can have unpleasant side effects, including diarrhea and cramping.

Diarrhea can lead to severe pain, dehydration, and electrolyte imbalances.

Researchers have concluded that the side effects caused by unpurified aloe vera juice are a result of the presence of anthraquinone, which is considered a laxative.

Though anthraquinone is an organic compound naturally found in the leaf of the aloe vera plant, it's considered toxic and should be avoided.

One 2013 studyTrusted Source found that aloe vera whole-leaf extract increased the risk of colon adenomas (benign) and carcinomas (cancer) in rats. However, another study on rats that same year noted that purified and decolorized juice is a safer option when compared to colored aloe vera.

When shopping, look for the following statements on the label:

- purified
- decolorized
- organic
- safety tested

2.AMAZING USES FOR ALOE VERA

1. Heals burns

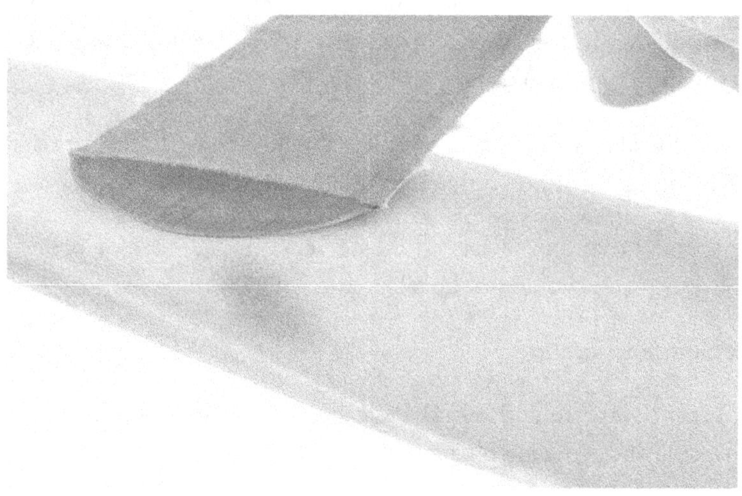

Due to its soothing, moisturizing, and cooling properties, aloe vera is often used to treat burns.

A 2013 studyTrusted Source with 50 participants found that people who used aloe vera gel to treat superficial and partial thickness burns showed better results than the group that used a 1 percent silver sulfadiazine cream.

The aloe vera group showed earlier wound healing and pain relief. Plus, aloe vera had the benefit of being inexpensive.

More research is needed, but the available evidenceTrusted Source suggests that aloe gel can be beneficial for burn wound healing.

If you have a sunburn or another mild burn, apply aloe vera a few times a day to the area. If you have a severe burn, seek medical help before applying aloe.

2. Improves digestive health

Consuming aloe vera may benefit your digestive tract and help to soothe and cure stomach ailments, including irritable bowel syndrome (IBS).

A 2018 review looked at three studies with 151 people. Results from the studies showed that aloe vera significantly improved symptoms of IBS when compared to a placebo. No adverse effects were reported, though more research is needed using a larger study size.

Additionally, aloe vera may help inhibit the growth of H. pylori bacteria, which is found in your digestive tract and can lead to ulcers.

Keep in mind that this advice is for aloe vera only. Other aloe plants may be poisonous and should not be taken internally.

3. Promotes oral health

Aloe vera toothpaste and mouthwash are natural options for improving oral hygiene and reducing plaque.

Results of a 2017 studyTrusted Source found that people who used an aloe vera toothpaste showed significant improvements to their oral health.

The study included 40 adolescents who were divided into two groups. Each group used either an aloe vera toothpaste or a traditional toothpaste containing triclosan twice daily.

After 30 days, the aloe toothpaste was found to be more effective than the triclosan toothpaste in lowering levels of candida, plaque, and gingivitis.

People who used the aloe vera toothpaste showed better overall oral health without experiencing any adverse effects.

4. Clears acne

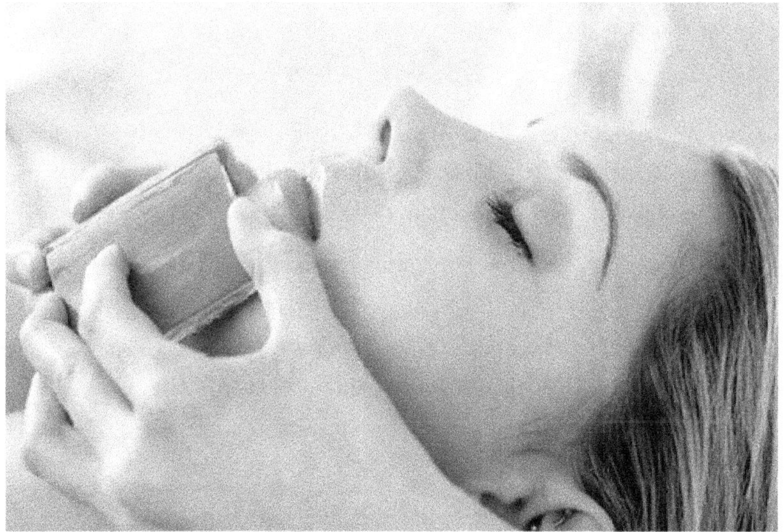

Using fresh aloe on your face may help clear up acne. You can also purchase aloe products designed for acne, including cleansers, toners, and creams. These may have the extra benefit of containing other effective ingredients, too.

Acne products made with aloe may be less irritating to the skin than traditional acne treatments.

A small 2014 study found that a cream combining conventional acne medication with aloe vera gel was significantly more effective than acne medication alone or a placebo in treating mild to moderate acne.

In this study, improvements were seen in lower levels of inflammation and fewer lesions in the group who used the combination cream over a period of eight weeks.

5. Natural Skincare

The use of aloe vera in skincare is no surprise as it's a well known plant that has been a successful, effective skincare ingredient for a long time.

The plant offers great benefits for the skin and hair and its properties have been recognised for thousands of years in traditional medicine; its use has been recorded as early as 2,200 BC, and is associated with important historical characters such as Cleopatra and Alexander the Great.

As a cosmetic ingredient, aloe vera is widely used in many mainstream skincare and cosmetics' products. The plant is very skin-friendly and has a low risk of causing allergies, sensitivity or skin reactions, and it is also versatile.

It is common in after-sun products, and in facial, hair and body care. Aloe vera is also a popular plant for scientific research with many studies being conducted to investigate its properties and composition.

Uses of Aloe Vera in Skincare

Among Aloe vera's active components, we have lipophilic and hydro-soluble vitamins, minerals, enzymes, simple and complex polysaccharides, phenolic compounds and organic acids, which together are responsible for its properties.

Aloe vera leaves have two distinct parts: the outer green peel; and the inner colorless gel. Just be careful not to confuse the bitter yellow liquid (exudate) from the outer peel with the clear inner gel.

Both parts have different components and activities so it's very important to distinguish between them and choose the appropriate part of the aloe vera plant depending on the properties you intend to add to your cosmetic.

Aloe Vera Gel

Aloe vera gel has great moisturising properties. That's because it is rich in polysaccharides, which also give it a gel-like appearance.

The polysaccharides are highly hygroscopic (water-loving) and bind to moisture. On the other hand, its structure forms a protective film for the skin, which helps give it its healing properties. It also aids protection of the epidermis and the skin's ability to restore itself.

Some studies point to possible analgesic and anti-inflammatory activities of the gel; properties that would be particularly beneficial on skin wounds, burns and promotion of radiation damage repair. Aloe vera gel also comprises vitamins, amino acids, minerals and enzymes, which provide its skin-soothing effect.

Aloe vera leaf exudate

The leaf exudate, which originates in aloe vera's green peel has been studied for both toxic and medicinal properties. Researchers are working on isolating the components present in the exudate, with a view to its application in both medicinal and cosmetic products.

The exudate's composition varies in different species.

However, it invariably contains several components that cause skin irritation and erythema (redness): phenolic compounds, particularly chromone, anthraquinone or anthrone derivatives are often the cause.

For this reason, we recommend that you use only aloe vera gel in your formulations, and avoid the leaf exudate.

Another component of interest in aloe vera leaf exudate is aloin, which has been isolated and studied for its skin-lightening properties with great results.

Here, we've compiled the components that make aloe vera an appealing ingredient to work with:

Useful Properties of Aloe Vera in Skincare	
Advantages:	<ul><li>Easy to find</li><li>Low price</li><li>Effective</li><li>Skin-friendly</li></ul>
Key Properties:	<ul><li>Moisturising</li><li>Skin Soothing</li><li>Analgesic and anti-inflammatory</li><li>Damage repair</li></ul>
Components:	<ul><li>Lipophilic and hydrosoluble vitamins</li><li>Minerals</li><li>Enzymes</li><li>Simple and complex polysaccharides</li><li>Phenolic compounds</li><li>Organic acids</li></ul>
Ingredients:	<ul><li>Aloe vera powder</li><li>Aloe vera gel</li><li>Aloe vera oil – infused</li><li>Aloe vera glycerite</li></ul>

6. Relieves anal fissures

If you have anal fissures, applying an aloe vera cream to the affected area several times throughout the day may help promote healing.

A 2014 studyTrusted Source found that using a cream containing aloe vera juice powder was effective in treating chronic anal fissures. People used the aloe cream three times a day for six weeks.

Improvements were shown in pain, hemorrhaging upon defection, and wound healing. These results were significantly different from those of the control group. While this research is promising, further studies are needed to expand upon this research.

7.Heartburn relief

Gastroesophageal reflux disease (GERD) is a digestive disorder that often results in heartburn. A 2010 review suggested that consuming 1 to 3 ounces of aloe gel at mealtime could reduce the severity of GERD. It may also ease other digestion-related problems. The plant's low toxicity makes it a safe and gentle remedy for heartburn.

8.Keeping produce fresh

A 2014 study published online by the Cambridge University Press looked at tomato plants coated with aloe gel. The report showed evidence that the coating successfully blocked the growth of many types of harmful bacteria on the vegetables.

Similar results were found in a different study with apples. This means that aloe gel could help fruits and vegetables stay fresh, and eliminate the need for dangerous chemicals that extend the shelf life of produce.

9.Lowering your blood sugar

Ingesting two tablespoons of aloe vera juice per day can cause blood sugar levels to fall in people with type 2 diabetes, according to a studyTrusted Source in Phytomedicine: International Journal of Phytotherapy and Phytopharmacy. This could mean that aloe vera may have a future in diabetes treatment. These results were confirmed by another studyTrusted Source published in Phytotherapy Research that used pulp extract.

But people with diabetes, who take glucose-lowering medications, should use caution when consuming aloe vera. The juice along with diabetes medications could possibly lower your glucose count to dangerous levels.

10.A natural laxative

Aloe vera is considered a natural laxative. A handful of studies have looked into the benefits of the succulent to aid digestion. The results appear to be mixed.

A team of Nigerian scientists conducted a study on rats and found that gel made from typical aloe vera houseplants was able to relieve constipation.

But another study by the National Institutes of Health looked at the consumption of aloe vera whole-leave extract. Those findings revealed tumor growth in the large intestines of laboratory rats.

In 2002, the U.S. Food and Drug Administration required that all over-the-counter aloe laxative products be removed from the U.S. market or be reformulated.

The Mayo Clinic recommends that aloe vera can be used to relieve constipation, but sparingly. They advise that a dose of 0.04 to 0.17 grams of dried juice is sufficient.

If you have Crohn's disease, colitis, or hemorrhoids you shouldn't consume aloe vera. It can cause severe abdominal cramps and diarrhea. You should stop taking aloe vera if you're taking other medications. It may decrease your body's ability to absorb the drugs

11.Aloe vera benefits for your hair

Calms an itchy scalp

Seborrheic dermatitis is the clinical term for the condition we call dandruff. The symptoms of an itchy scalp and flaking skin under your hair can be treated with aloe vera.

A 1998 study found that aloe vera helped resolve the scalp inflammation that dandruff causes. The fatty acids found in the aloe plant have anti-inflammatory properties.

Deep cleans oily hair

Aloe vera cleanses the hair follicle efficiently, stripping off extra sebumTrusted Source (oil) and residue from other hair products. But aloe vera doesn't hurt your hair strands while it cleans. Unlike other chemicals in hair products, aloe vera is gentle and preserves the integrity of your hair.

Using aloe vera is a great way to get hair that looks healthier, shinier, and softer.

Strengthens and repairs hair strands

Aloe vera containsTrusted Source vitamins A, C, and E. All three of these vitamins contribute to cell turnover, promoting healthy cell growth and shiny hair. Vitamin B-12 and folic acid are also containedTrusted Source in aloe vera gel. Both of these components can keep your hair from falling out.

Aloe vera is a popular product that people use on their skin after sun exposure. This is because of its high collagen content and cooling properties. The vitamin content in aloe vera suggests that it might work to repair sun damage to your hair, too.

Promotes hair growth

Aloe vera has the incredible ability to increase blood circulationTrusted Source to an area. That's part of why its healing properties are so unique.

When you use aloe vera on your hair and scalp, blood flow to your scalp increases. When your scalp has been cleansed and your hair has been conditioned with aloe vera, you might see that hair breakage and loss slows down.

There are plenty of people who claim that aloe vera actually causes hair to grow much faster. But as of now, there's little clinical evidence to prove or disprove those claims.

Risks and warnings for aloe vera

There's usually little cause for concern when using aloe vera gel, but some people are allergic to it. Before using aloe vera topically, do a patch test. Rub a small bit of aloe vera on the inside of your wrist and wait up to two hours to see if your skin reacts poorly. This will let you know if you have an aloe sensitivity.

You should also be careful with topical aloe if you're using hydrocortisone cream on your skin. Aloe vera can increase the amount of cortisone that's absorbed by your skin when the two are used together.

Is aloe vera safe?

It's safe for most people to use aloe vera topically for minor skin care concerns. Generally, it's well tolerated, though skin irritations and allergic reactions are possible. Never use aloe vera or any severe cuts or burns.

Pay attention to how your body reacts to aloe. Notice if you experience any sensitivities or adverse reactions. Don't use aloe if you're allergic to garlic, onions, or tulips. Avoid taking aloe vera within two weeks of any scheduled surgery.

Women who are pregnant or breastfeeding, and children under the age of 12, should avoid the oral use of aloe vera.

Carefully follow the dosage information when taking aloe vera gel or latex internally. Limit your use to small periods of time. After a few weeks of use, take a break for at least one week. Always buy from a reputable brand to ensure safety and quality.

The laxative effect of aloe vera latex has the potential to cause diarrhea and abdominal cramps. These effects could inhibit the absorption of oral drugs and reduce their effectiveness.

Do not take aloe vera internally if you have the following conditions:

- hemorrhoids
- kidney conditions
- renal disorder
- cardiac condition
- Crohn's disease
- ulcerative colitis
- intestinal obstruction
- diabetes

Possible side effects of aloe vera include:

- kidney issues
- blood in the urine
- low potassium
- muscle weakness
- diarrhea
- nausea or stomach pain
- electrolyte imbalances

Talk to your doctor before using aloe vera if you are also taking the following medications, because aloe vera may interact with them:

- water pills(diuretics)
- herbs and supplements
- corticosteroids
- digoxin (Lanoxin)
- warfarin (Coumadin, Jantoven)
- sevoflurane (Ultane)
- stimulant laxatives
- diabetes medications
- anticoagulants

3.HOW TO CARE FOR ALOE VERA PLANTS

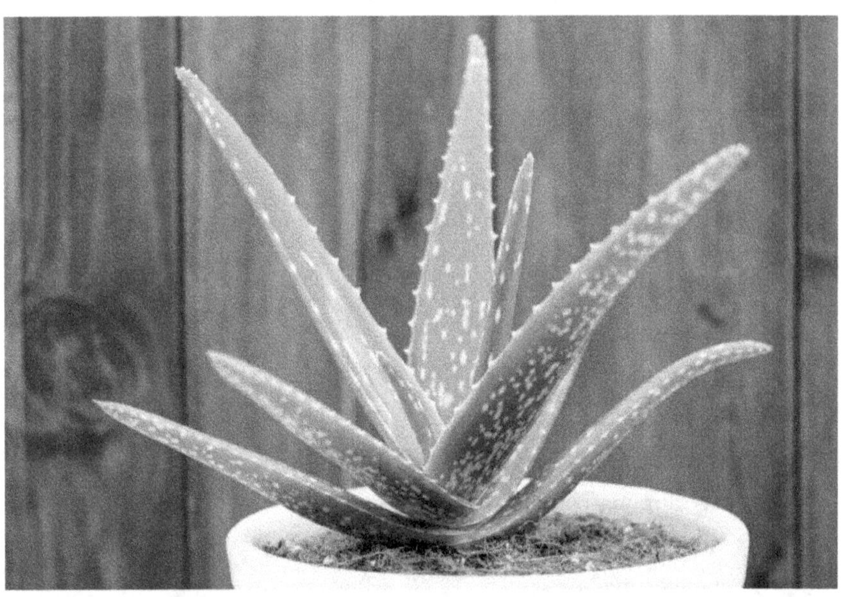

The **aloe vera** plant is an easy, attractive succulent that makes for a great indoor companion. Aloe vera plants are useful, too, as the juice from their leaves can be used to relieve pain from scrapes and burns when applied topically.

Here's how to grow and care for aloe vera plants in your home!

Aloe vera is a succulent plant species of the genus *Aloe*. The plant is stemless or very short-stemmed with thick, greenish, fleshy leaves that fan out from the plant's central stem. The margin of the leaf is serrated with small teeth.

Before you buy an aloe, note that you'll need a location that offers bright, indirect sunlight (or, artificial sunlight).

However, the plant doesn't appreciate sustained direct sunlight, as this tends to dry out the plant too much and turn its leaves yellow.

Keep the aloe vera plant in a pot near a kitchen window for periodic use but avoid having the sun's rays hit it directly.

Please note: The gel from aloe vera leaves can be used topically, but should not be ingested by people or pets. It can cause unpleasant symptoms such as nausea or indigestion and may even be toxic in larger quantities.

PLANTING

Before planting

- It's important to chose the right type of planter. A pot made from terra-cotta or a similarly porous material is recommended, as it will allow the soil to dry thoroughly between waterings and will also be heavy enough to keep the plant from tipping over. A plastic or glazed pot may also be used, though these will hold more moisture.

- When choosing a container, be sure to pick one that has at least one drainage hole in the bottom. This is key, as the hole will allow excess water to drain out.

- Select a container that's about as wide as it is deep. If your aloe plant has a stem, choose a container that is deep enough for you to plant the entire stem under the soil.

- Aloe vera plants are succulents, so use a well-draining **potting mix**, such as those made for cacti and succulents. Do not use soil. A good mix should contain perlite, lava rock, coarse sand, or all three. Aloe vera plants are hardy, but a lack of proper drainage can cause rot and wilting, which is easily the most common cause of death for this plant.

- A layer of gravel, clay balls, or any other "drainage" material in the bottom of the pot is not necessary. This only takes up space that the roots could otherwise be using. A drainage hole is drainage enough!

- (Optional) To encourage your aloe to put out new roots after planting, dust the stem of the plant with a rooting hormone powder. Rooting hormone can be found at a local garden center or hardware store, or online.

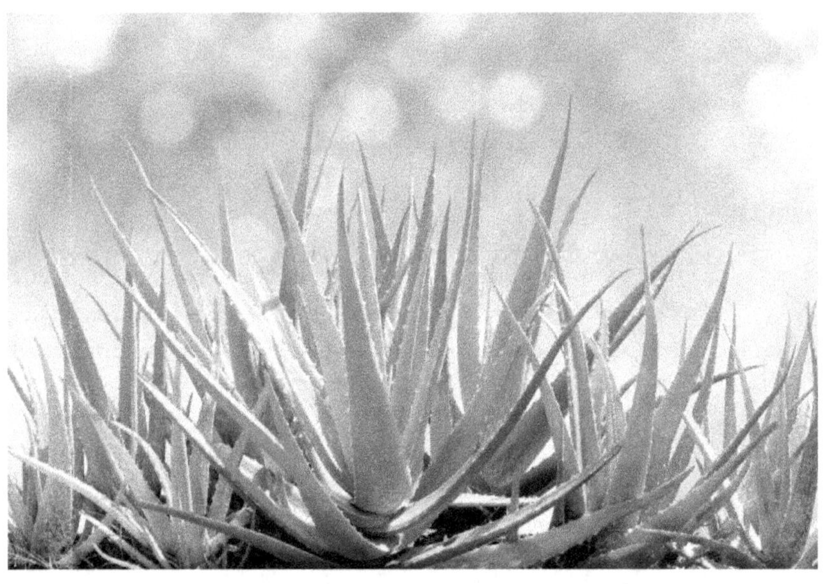

HOW TO PLANT (OR REPOT) AN ALOE VERA PLANT

If your aloe plant has grown leggy, has gotten too large, or simply needs an upgrade, it's time to repot it. Here's how:

1. **Prepare your pot.** After giving the new pot a quick rinse (or a good scrub, if it's a pot you've used before) and letting it dry thoroughly, place a small piece of screen over the drainage hole; this will keep the soil from falling out the bottom and will allow water to drain properly. A doubled-up piece of paper towel or newspaper can also work in a pinch, though these will break down over time.

2. **Prepare your plant.** Remove the aloe vera plant from its current pot and brush away any excess dirt from the roots, being careful not to damage the roots.

    o   If your plant has any pups, remove them now. (See the "Care" section of this page for instructions on removing and potting pups.)

    o   If your plant has a very long, spindly stem that won't fit in the pot, it is possible to trim the stem off partially. Note that this is risky and could kill the plant. To trim the stem: Cut off part of the stem, leaving as much as possible on the plant.

    o   Next, take the bare plant and place it in a warm area that gets indirect light. After several days, a callous will form over the wound. At this point, continue with the repotting instructions below.

3. **Plant your plant.** Fill the pot about a third of the way with a well-draining potting mix, then place your plant in the soil. Continue filling in soil around the plant, bearing in mind that you should leave at least ¾ of an inch of space between the top of the soil and the rim of the pot. The bottom leaves of the aloe plant should rest just above the soil, too. Do not water after planting.

4. **Ignore your plant (temporarily).** After you've placed your aloe in its new pot, don't water it for at least a week. This will decrease the chance of inducing rot and give the plant time to put out new

roots. Until the plant seems to be rooted and happy, keep it in a warm place that receives bright but indirect light.

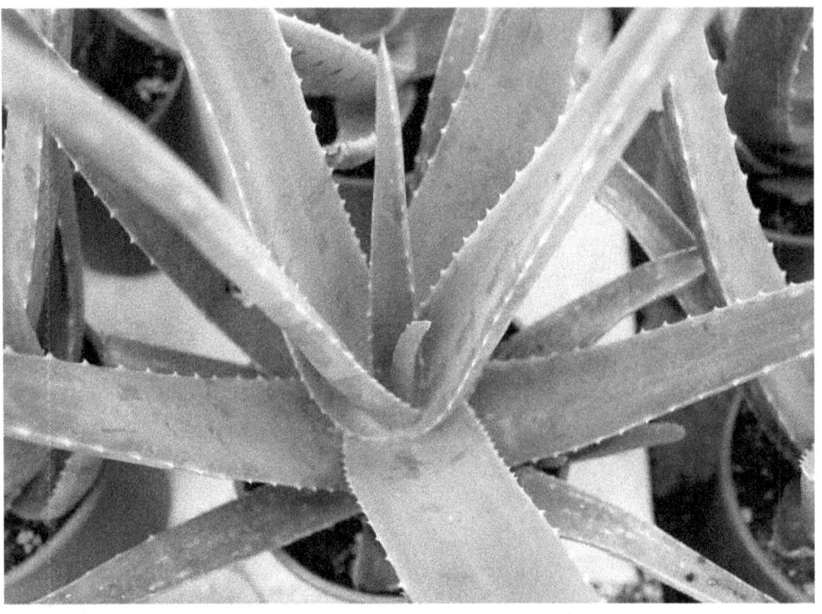

HOW TO CARE FOR AN ALOE VERA PLANT

- Place in bright, indirect sunlight or artificial light. A western or southern window is ideal. Aloe that are kept in low light often grow leggy.

- Aloe vera do best in temperatures between 55 and 80°F (13 and 27°C). The temperatures of most homes and apartment are ideal. From **May to September**, you can bring your plant outdoors without any problems, but do bring it back inside in the evening if nights are cold.

- Water aloe vera plants deeply, but infrequently. To discourage rot, allow the soil to dry at least 1 to 2 inches deep between waterings. Don't let your plant sit in water.

- Water about every 3 weeks and even more sparingly during the winter. Use your finger to test dryness before watering. If the potting mix stays wet, the plants' roots can begin to rot.

- Fertilize sparingly (no more than once a month), and only in the spring and summer with a balanced houseplant formula mixed at ½ strength.

- Repot when root bound, following the instructions given in "Planting," above.

REMOVING *&* REPLANTING ALOE VERA OFFSETS (PUPS)

Mature aloe vera plants often produce offsets—also known as plantlets, pups, or "babies"—that can be removed to produce an entirely new plant (a clone of the mother plant, technically).

1. Find where the offsets are attached to the mother plant and separate them using pruning shears, scissors, or a sharp knife. Leave at least an inch of stem on the offset.

2. Allow the offsets to sit out of soil for several days; this lets the offset form a callous over the cut, which helps to protect it from rot. Keep the offsets in a warm location with indirect light during this time.

3. Once the offsets have formed callouses, pot them in a standard succulent potting mix. The soil should be well-draining.

4. Put the newly-potted pups in a sunny location. Wait at least a week to water and keep the soil on the dry side.

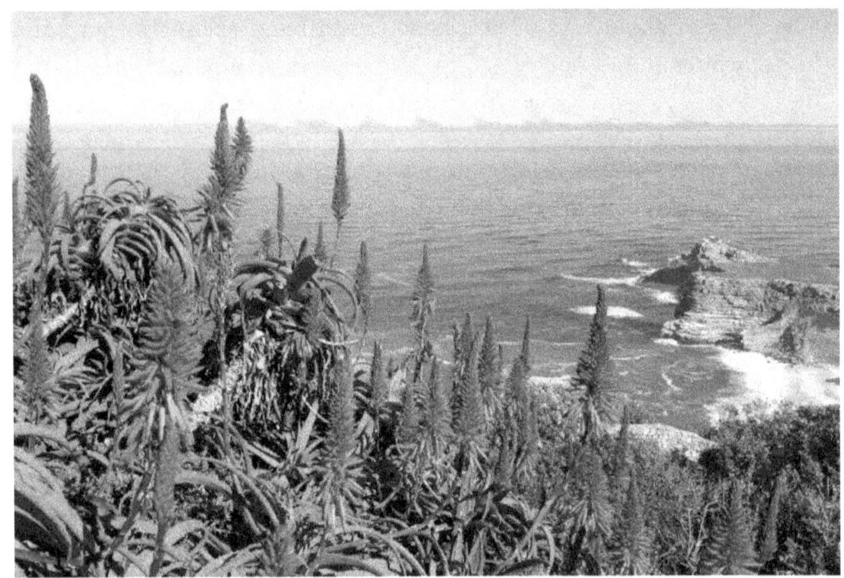

HOW TO GET YOUR ALOE VERA TO FLOWER

Mature aloe vera plants occasionally produce a tall flower spike—called an inflorescence—from which dozens of tubular yellow or red blossoms appear. This certainly adds another level of interest to the already lovely aloe!

Unfortunately, a bloom is rarely achievable with aloes that are kept as houseplants, since the plant requires nearly ideal conditions to produce flowers: lots of light, sufficient water, and the right temperature range.

Due to these requirements (mainly lighting), aloe flowers are usually only seen on plants grown outdoors year-round in warm climates.

To give your aloe the best shot at flowering:

- **Provide it with as much light as possible**, especially during spring and summer. Aloes can be kept outdoors in full sun during the summer, when temperatures are above 70°F (21°C). If nighttime temps threaten to drop below 60°F (16°C), bring the aloe inside.

- o **Note**: Don't move your aloe from indoors to full sun right away; it needs time to adjust to the intense light or it may sunburn. Allow it to sit in partial shade for about a week before moving it to a brighter location.

- **Make sure the plant is getting the right amount of water—** enough to keep it from drying out completely, but not enough to drown it! If the plant's being kept outdoors, make sure that it's not getting consistently soaked by summer rains.

- **Give your aloe a proper dormancy period in the fall and winter.** Aloe tend to bloom in late winter or early spring, so giving them a period of rest consisting of less frequent watering and cooler temperatures may encourage them to flower.

- **Don't be surprised if it still doesn't flower.** Despite our best efforts, indoor conditions just aren't ideal for most aloes, so don't be surprised if yours simply refuses to bloom!

PESTS/DISEASES

Aloe vera plants are most susceptible to the usual indoor plant pests, such as **mealybugs** and **scale**.

Common diseases include:

- **Root rot**

- **Soft rot**

- **Fungal stem rot**

- **Leaf rot**

Avoid overwatering to keep these conditions from developing or worsening.

ABOUT THE AUTHOR

I am Tammie Rowe. I'm a student in university. I've compiled a great list here and I've excited they're all in the one spot. I hope you enjoy it as much as I enjoyed making it!

When you finish this book it would be amazing if you could leave a review for me as it'd mean the world.

Thanks so much for reading by my little corner.

Hope you enjoy the book!